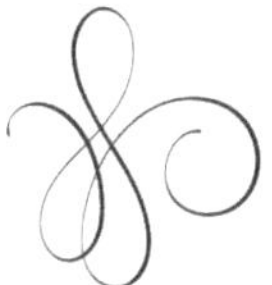

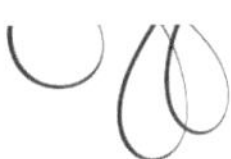

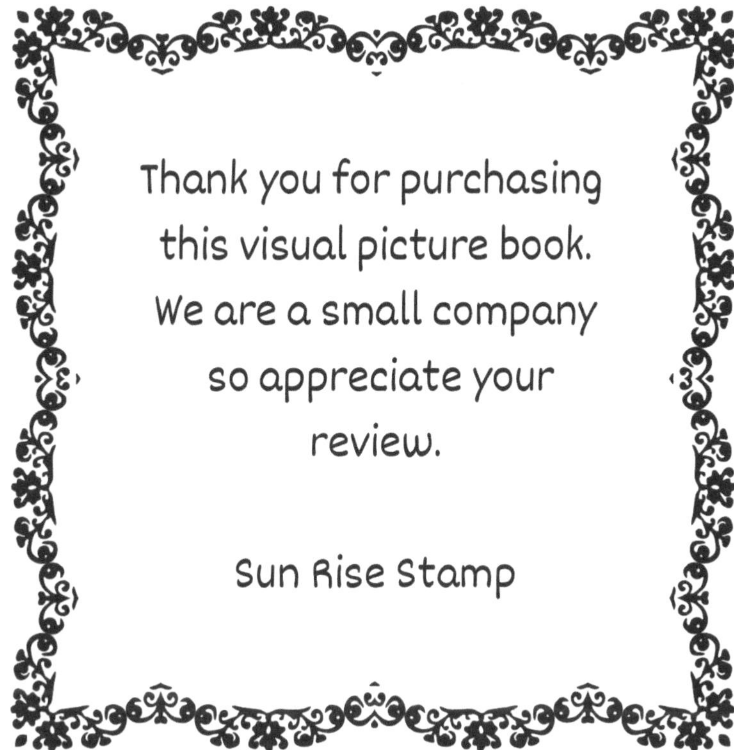

Thank you for purchasing
this visual picture book.
We are a small company
so appreciate your
review.

Sun Rise Stamp

The pictures in this book can be used for collage projects
cut out reminders or can be reviewed in book form

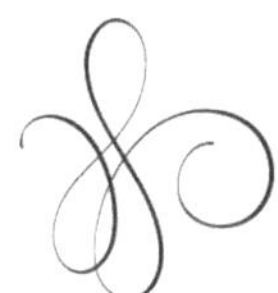

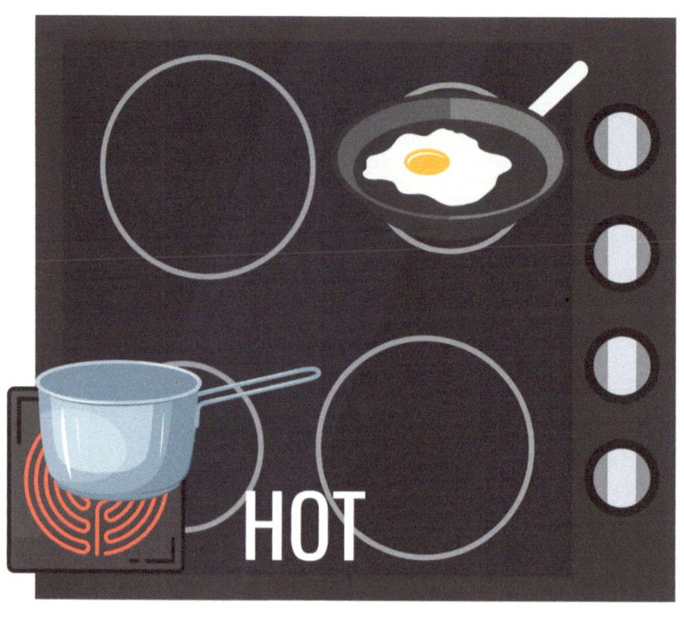

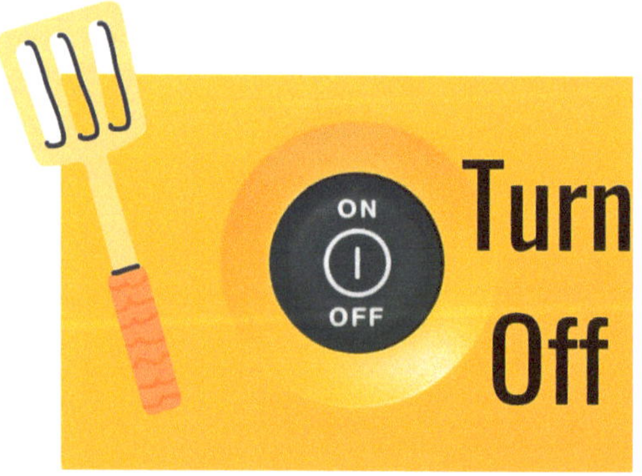

Turn Off Cooker after use

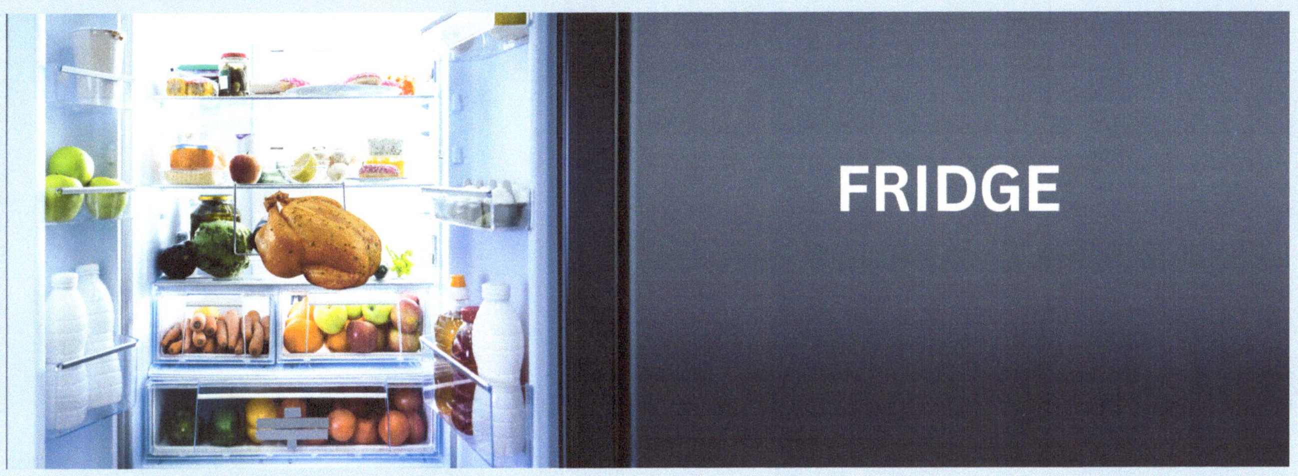
FRIDGE

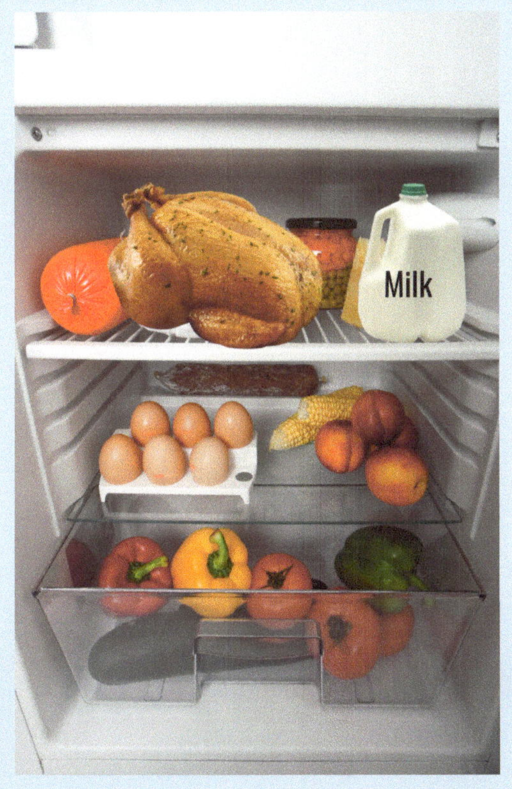
Milk

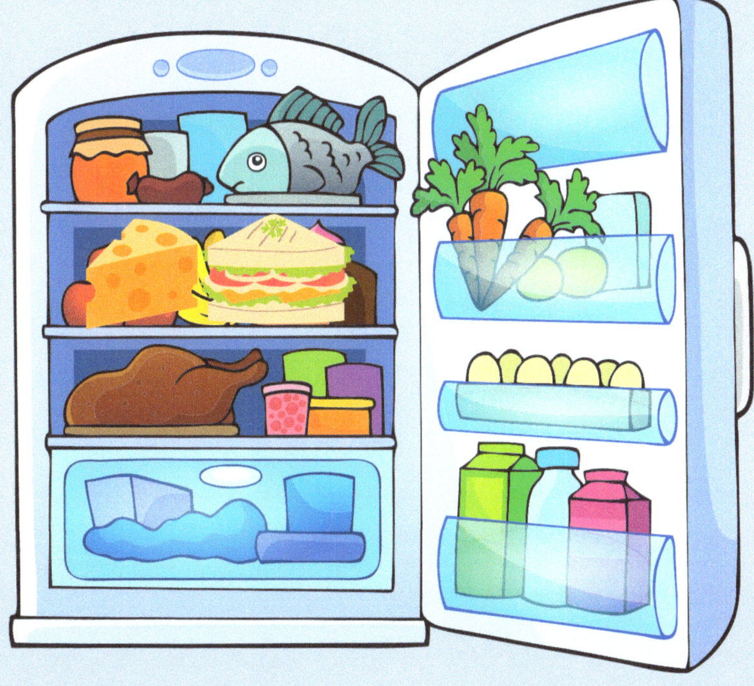

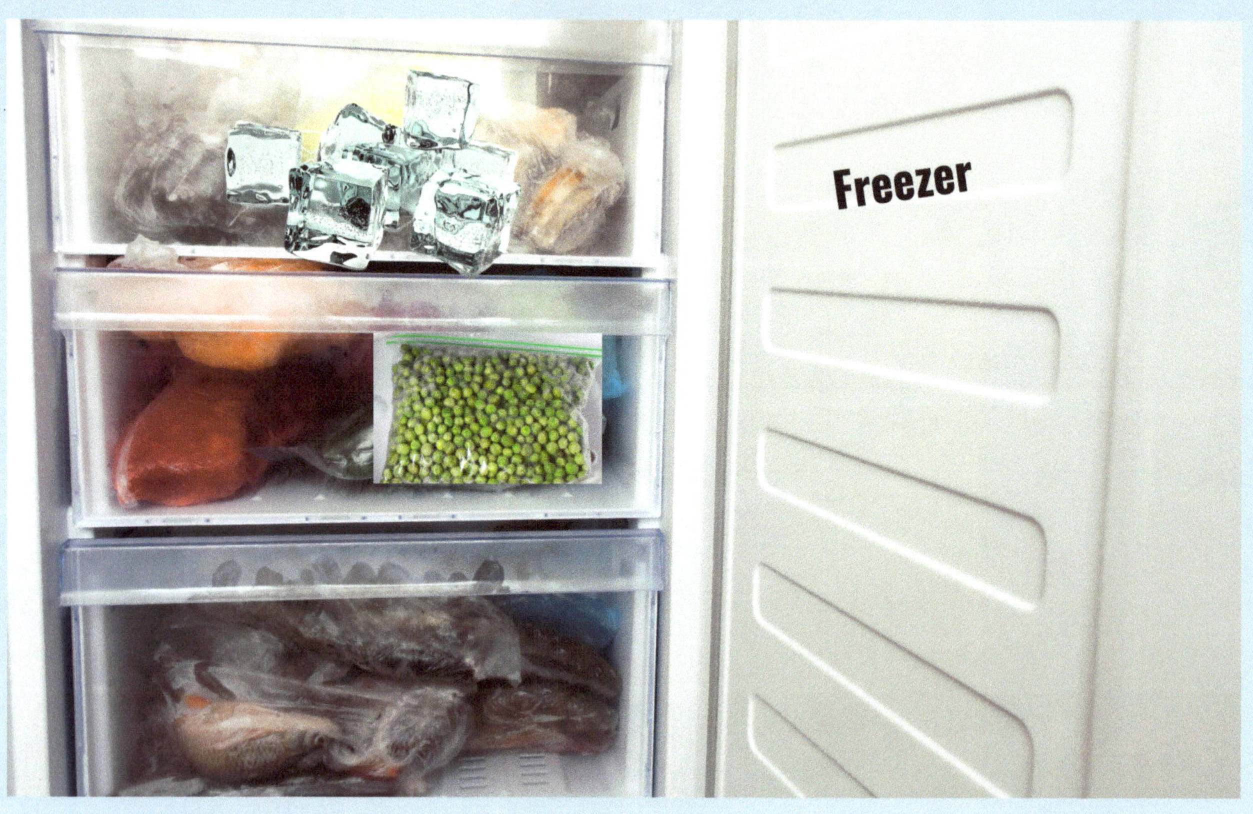

Defrost food before cooking

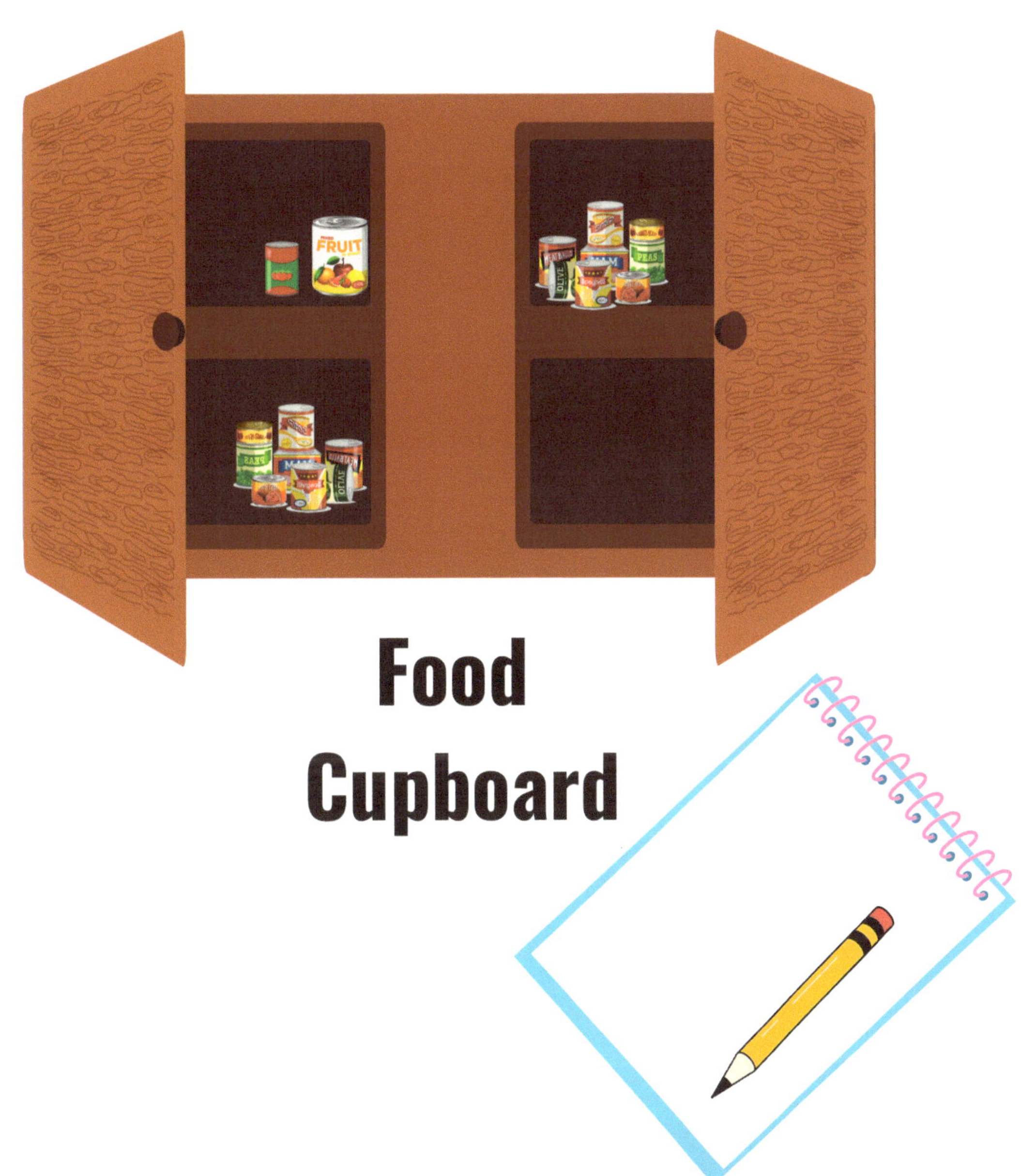

Food
Cupboard

Write a shopping list

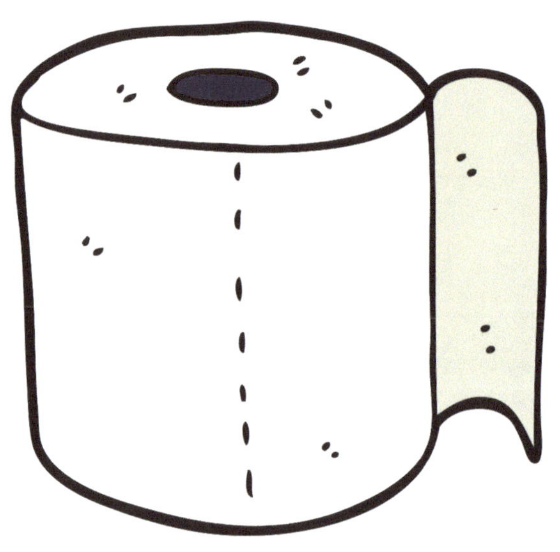

Buy loo roll often.

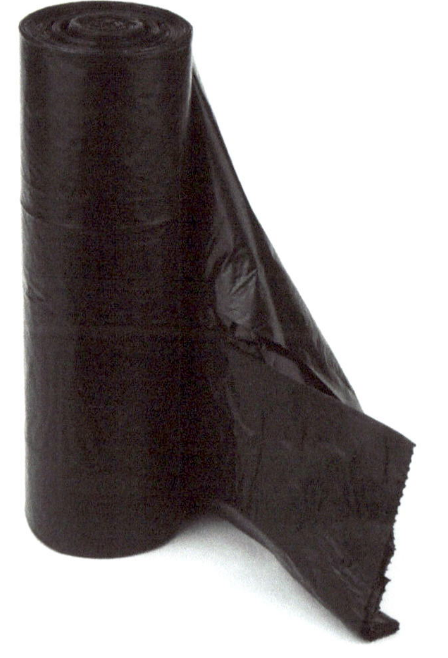

Buy bin liners often.

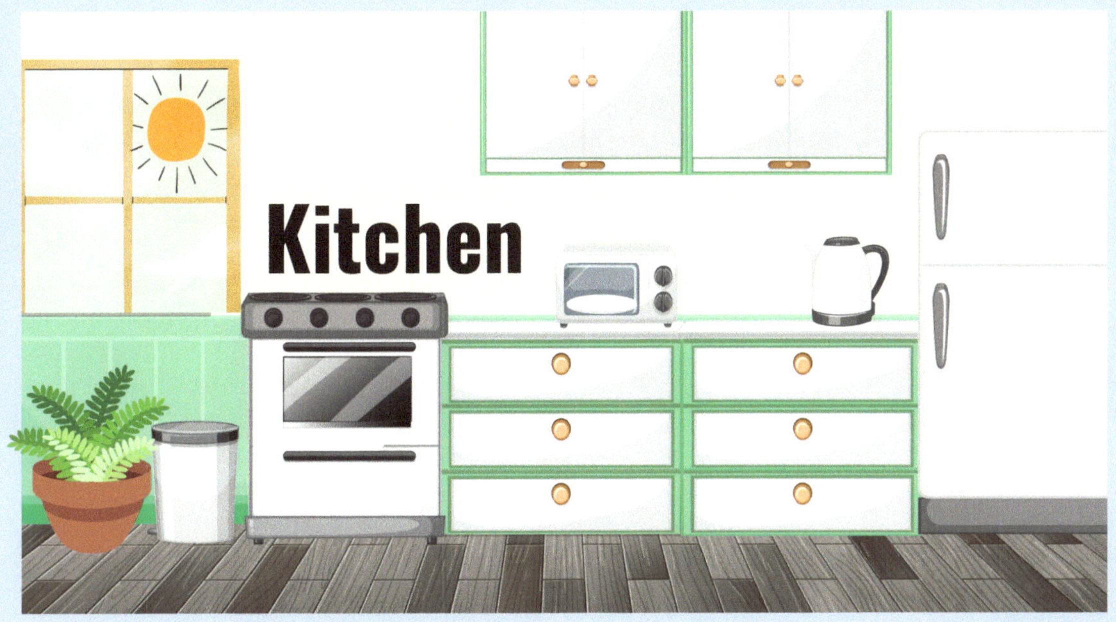

Kitchen

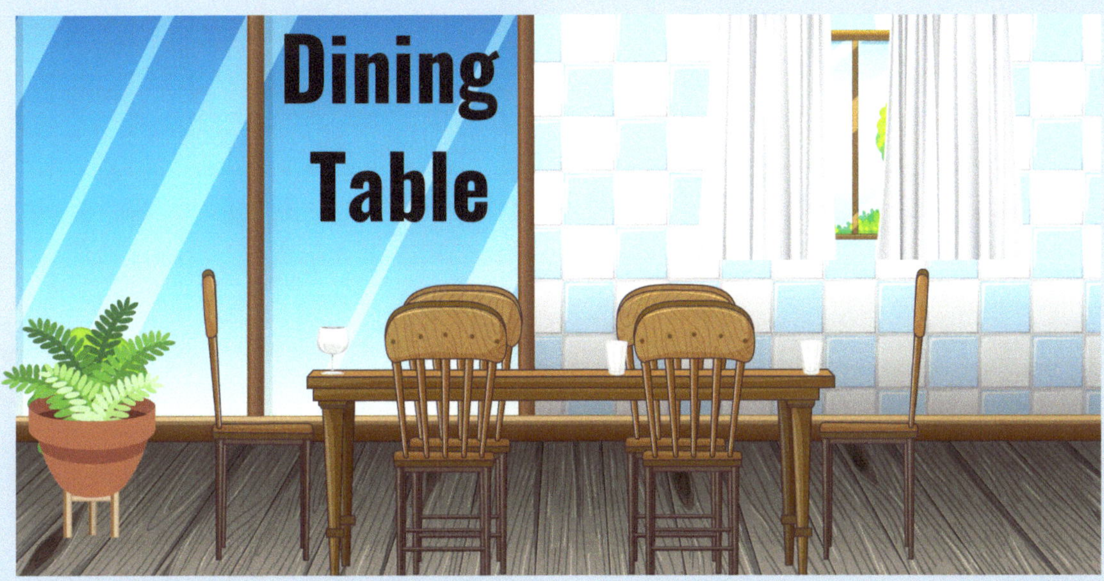

Dining
Table

MICROWAVE

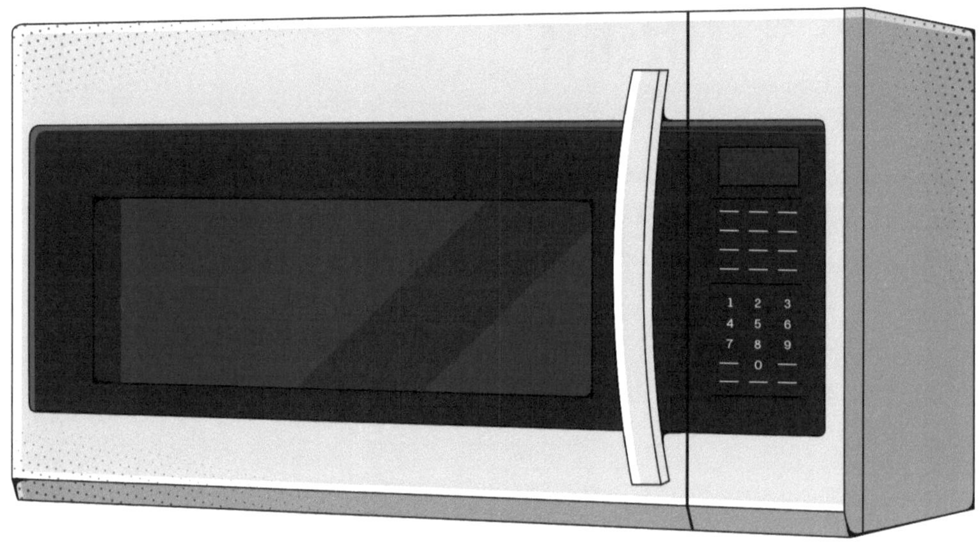

Heat Food Quickly.

KETTLE

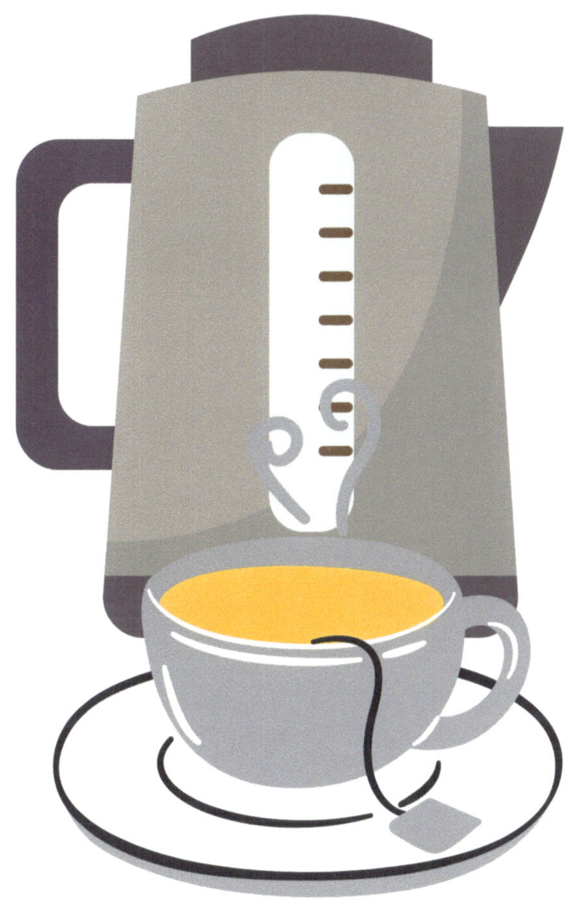

Hot Water For Drink

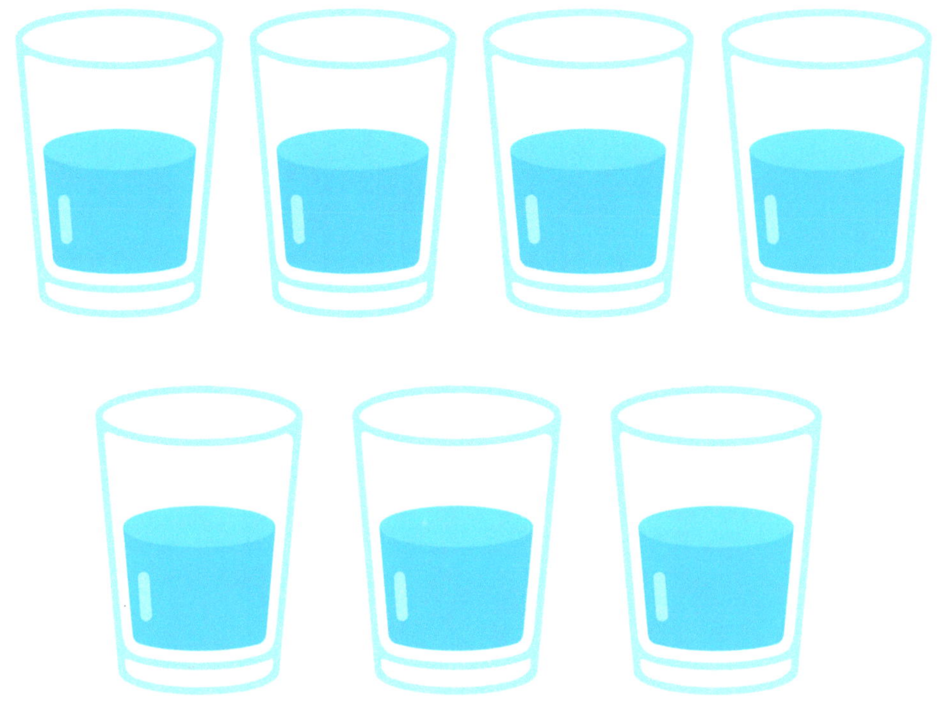

Drink Water Through Day.

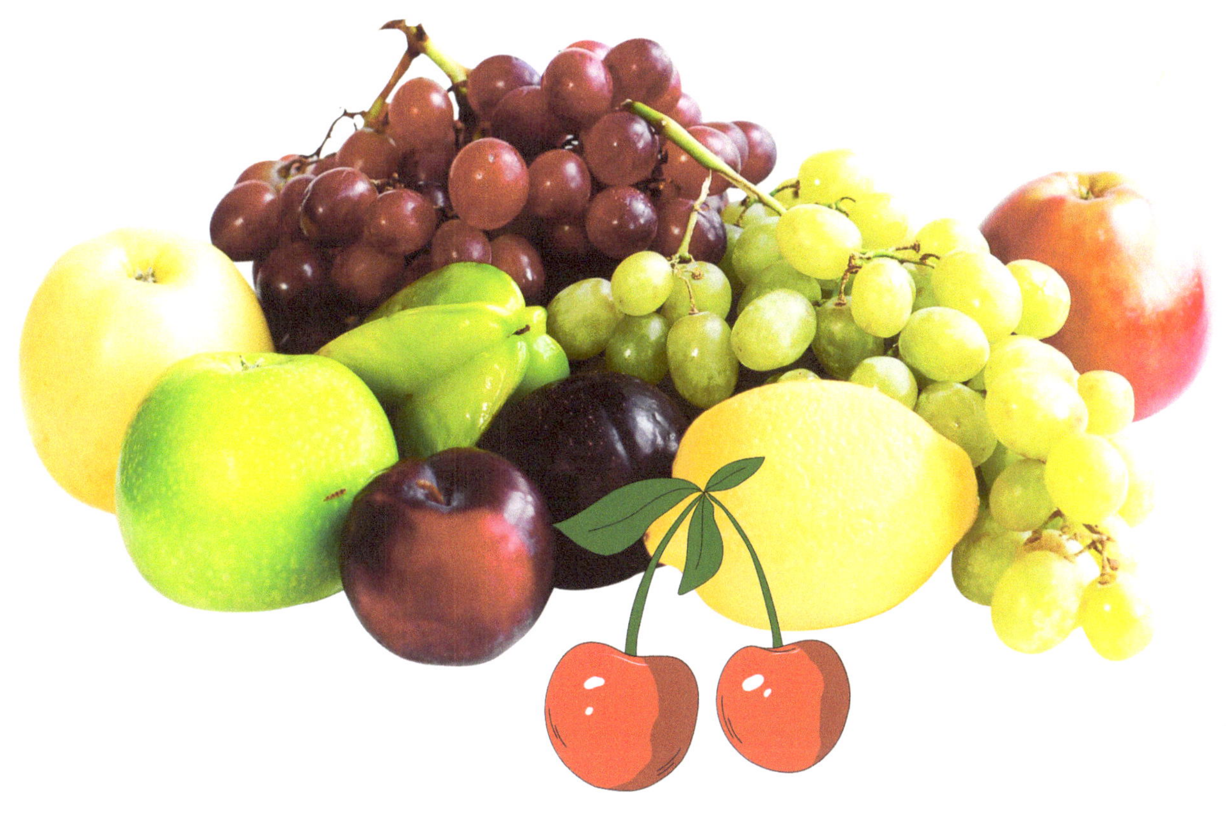

HEALTHY FOODS

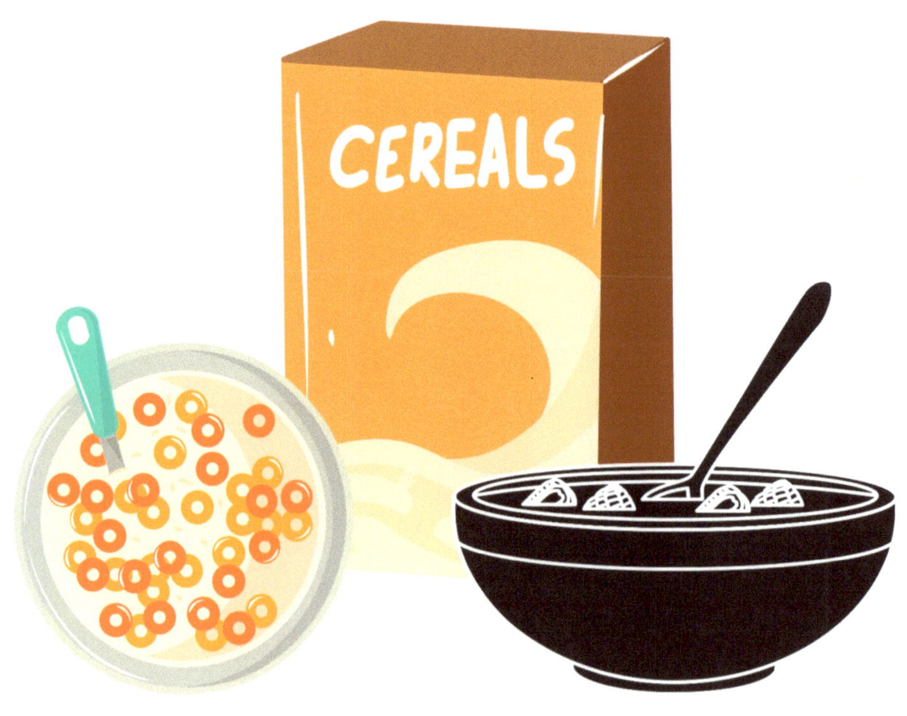

BREAKFAST

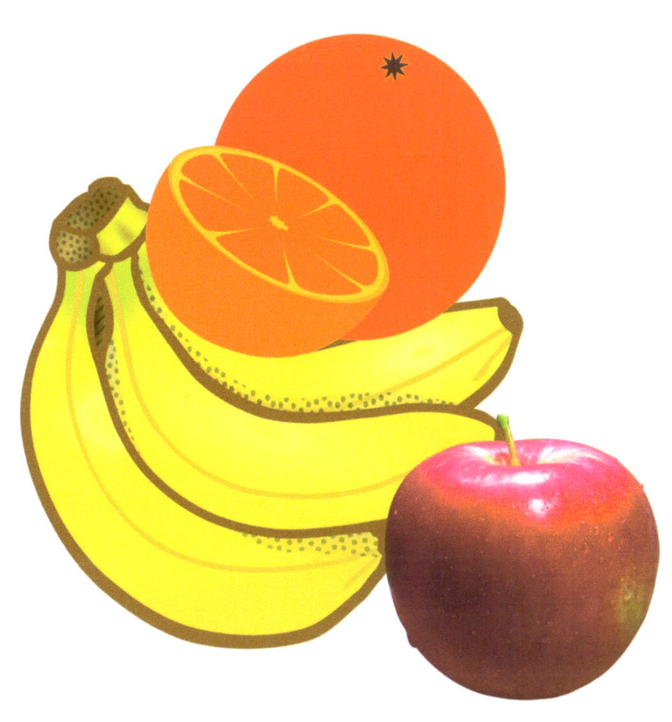

SNACKS

LUNCH

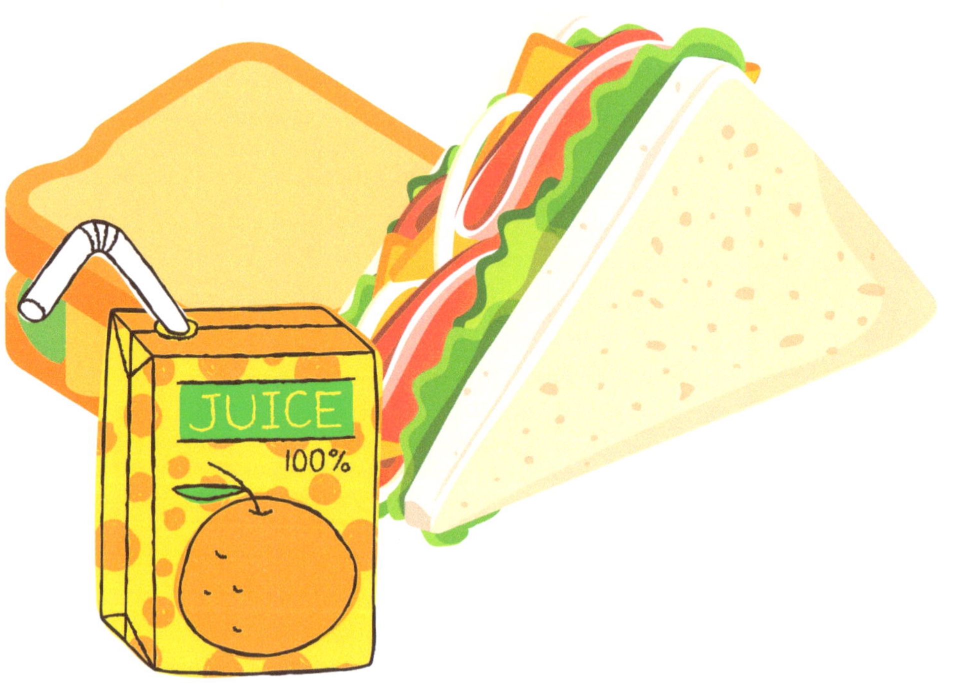

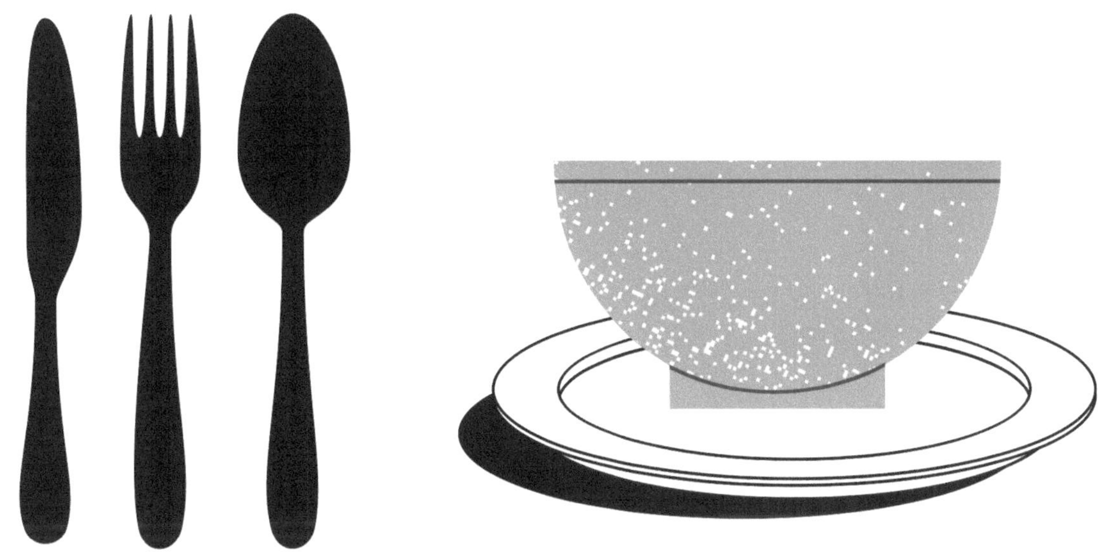

Cutlery and Crockery

DINNER

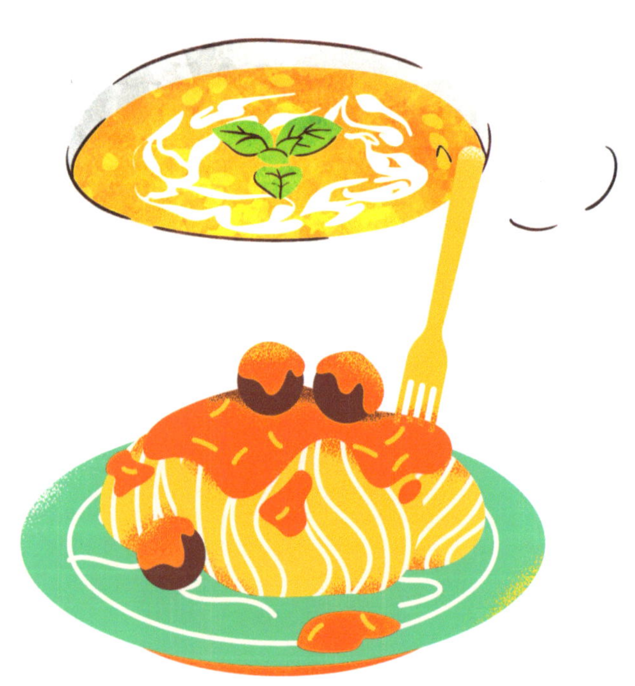

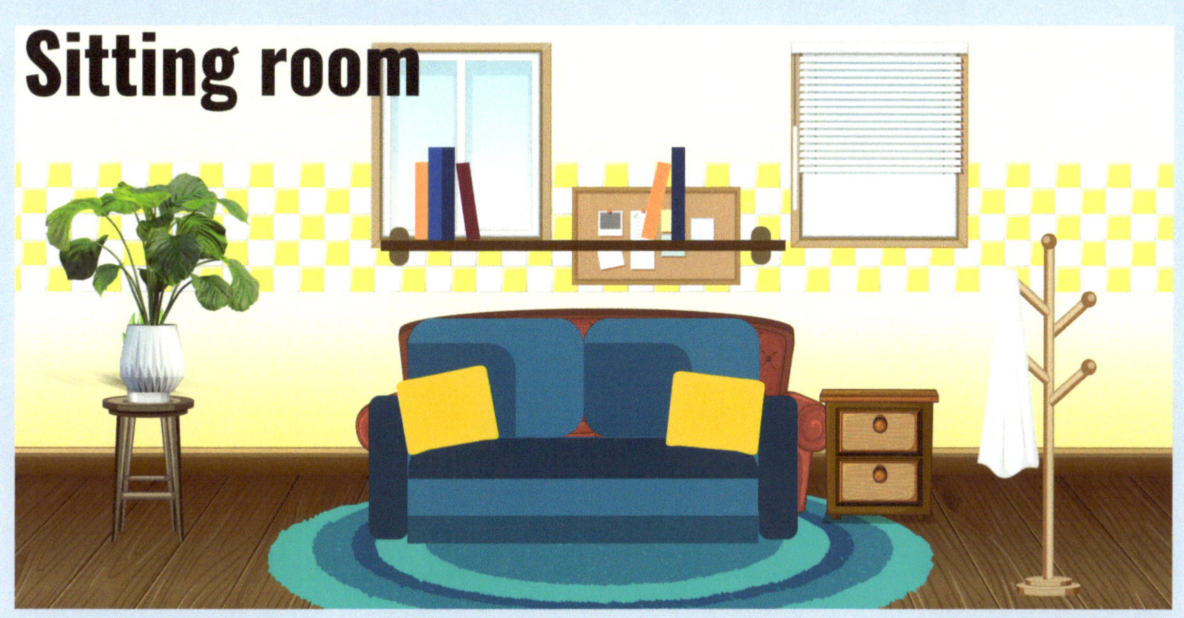
Sitting room

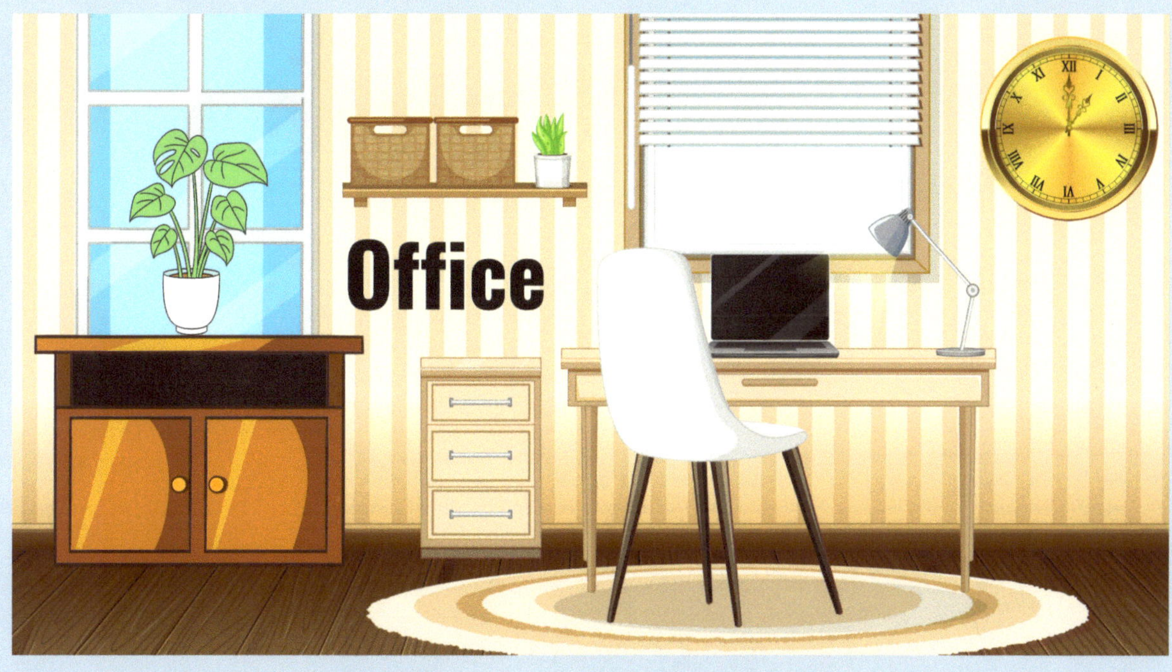
Office

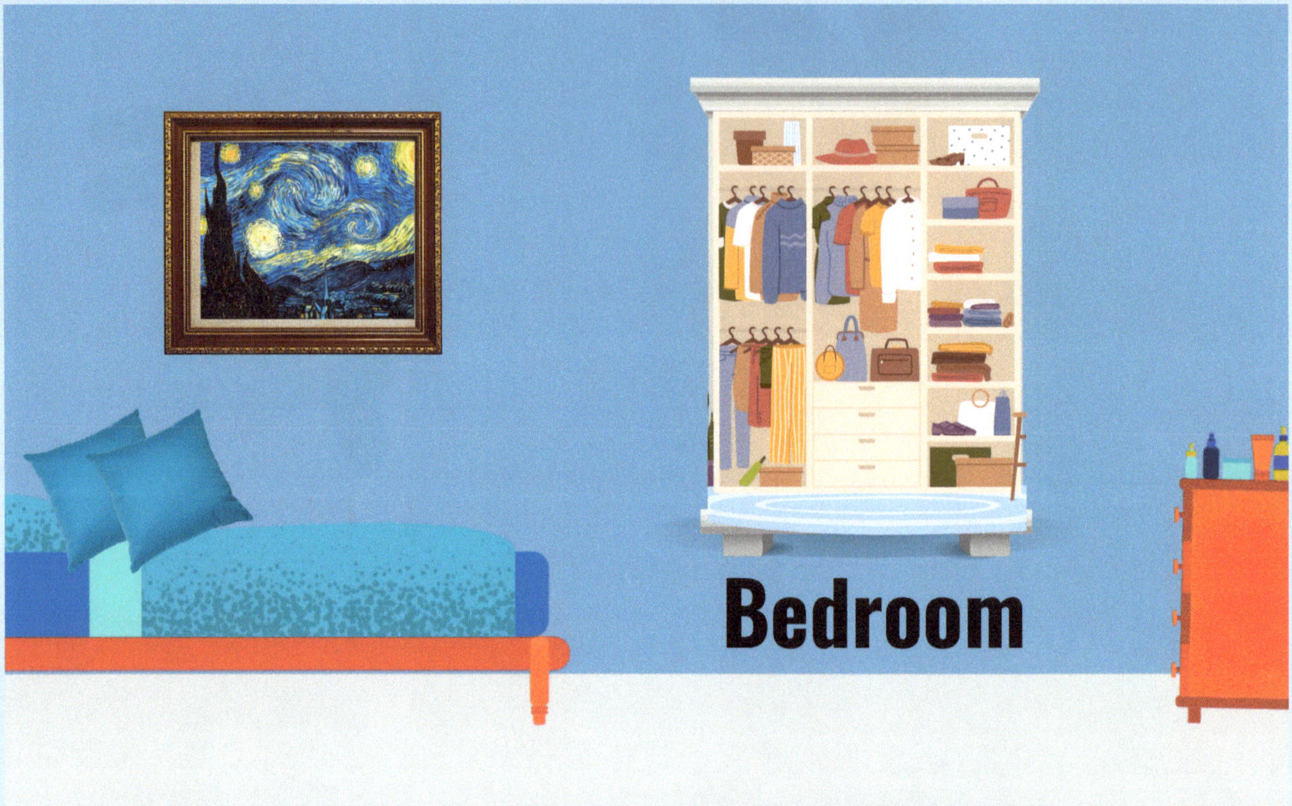

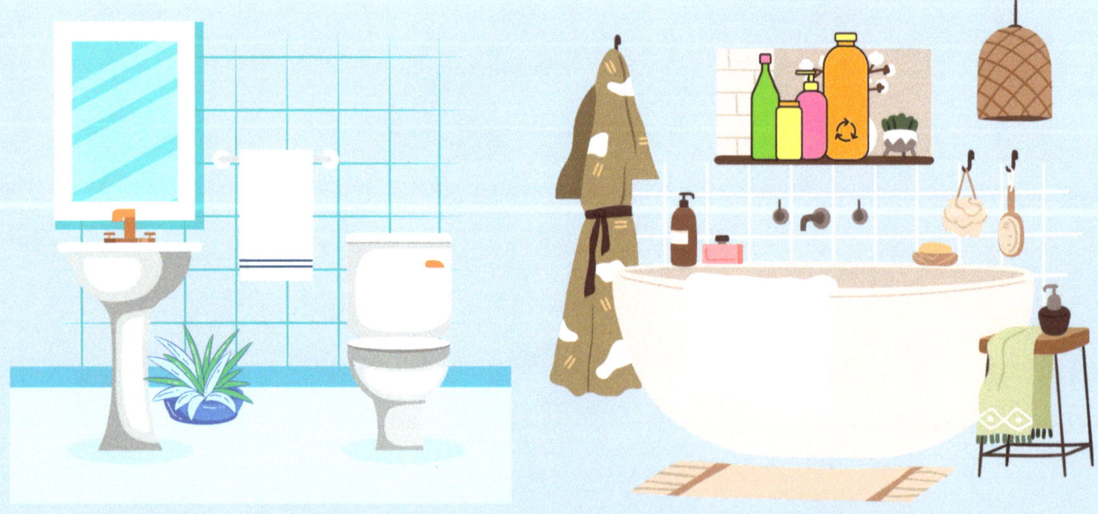

Bedroom
Bathroom

Wash Regularly

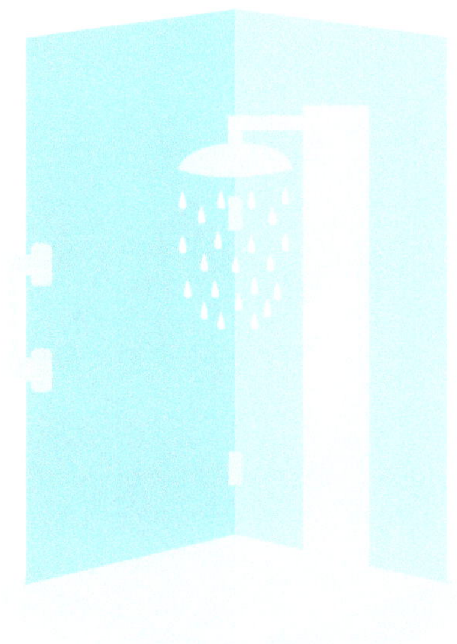

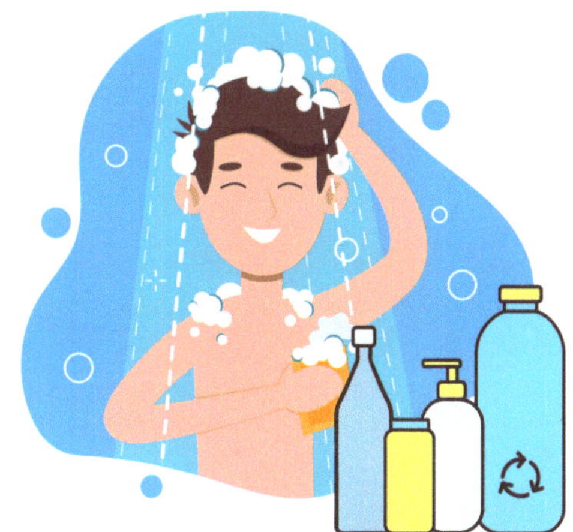

Wash off shampoo and shower gel

Use Towels to Dry

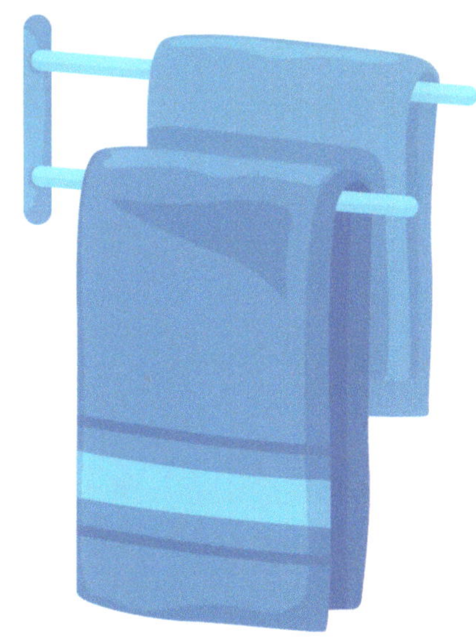

Brush teeth Twice a day

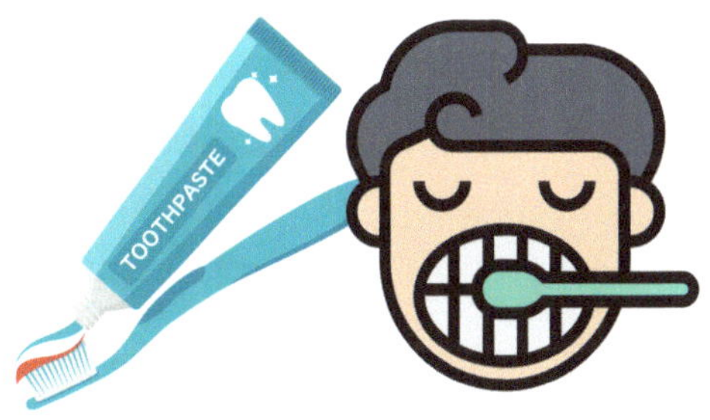

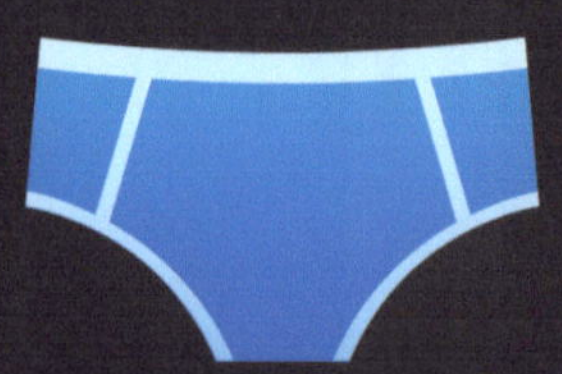

Monday

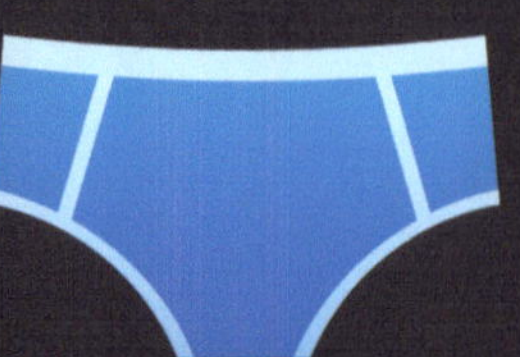

Tuesday

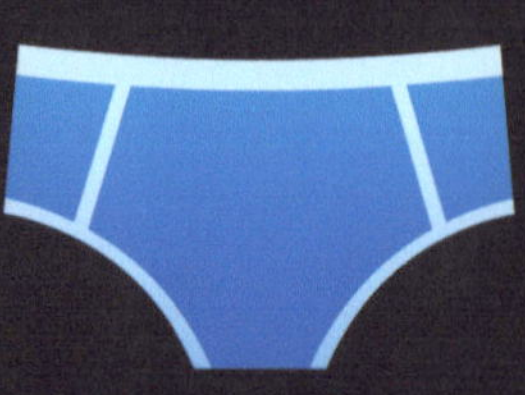

Wednesday

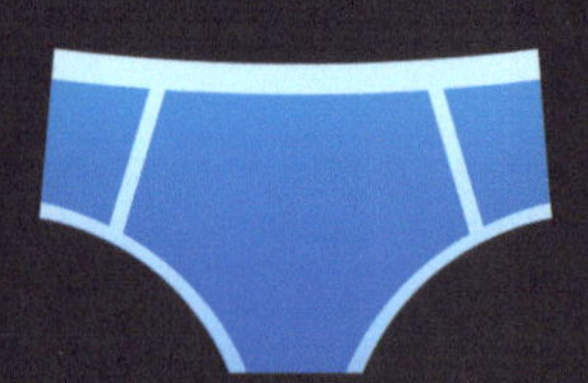

Thursday

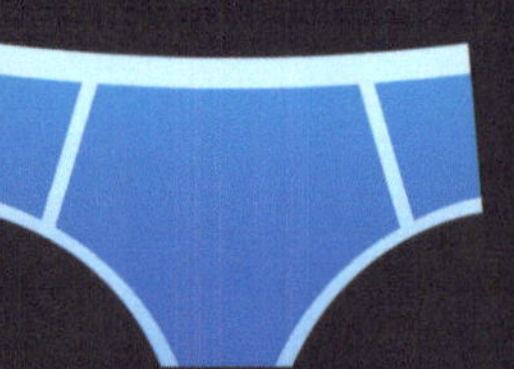

Friday

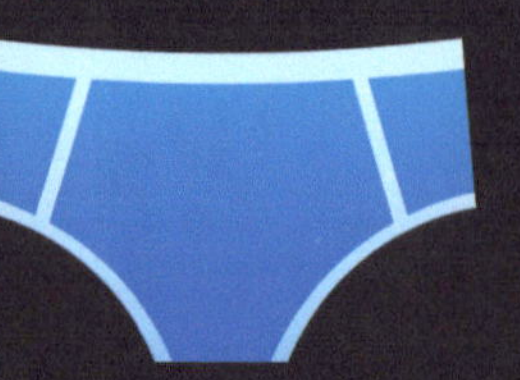

Saturday

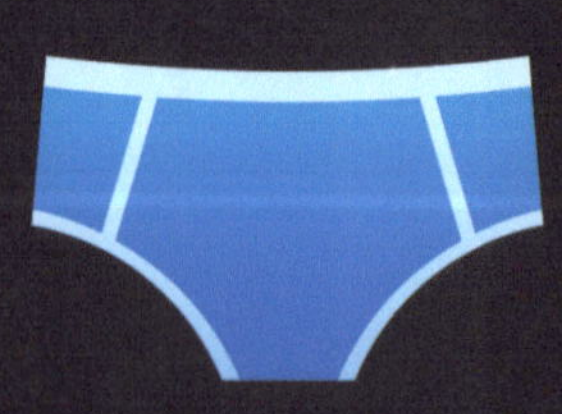

Sunday

NEW PANTS EVERYDAY

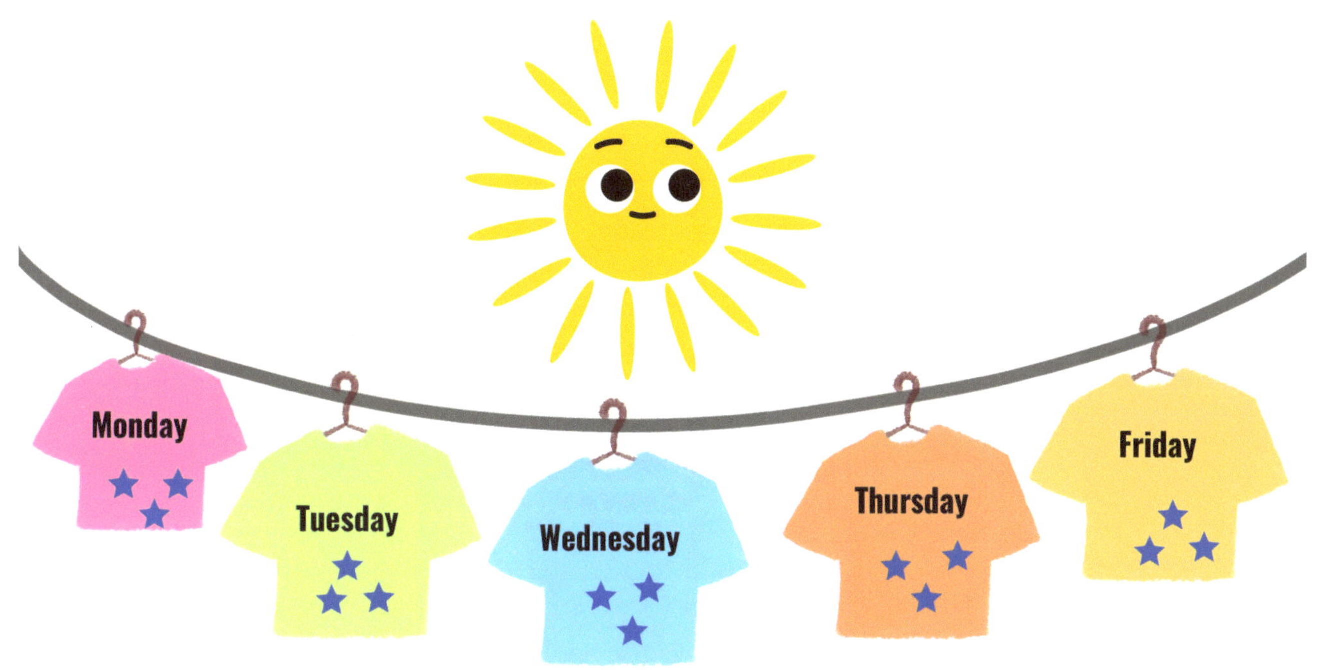

Clean Clothes for each day of the week

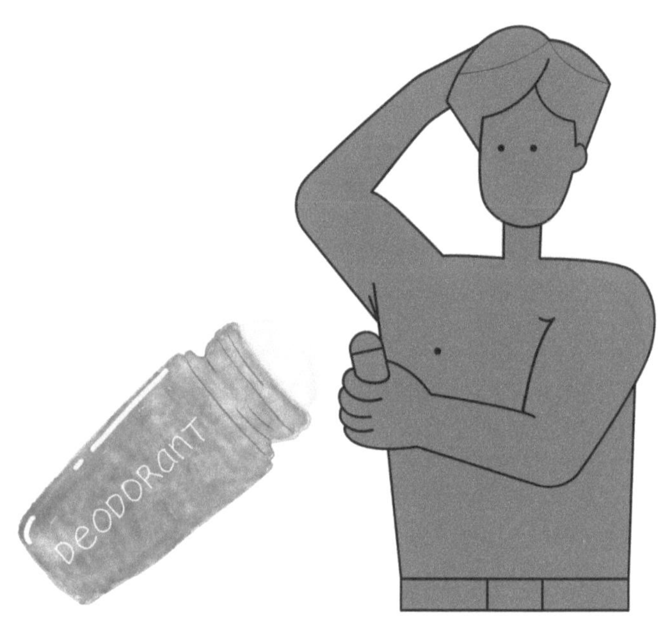

**Stay Fresh
Put Deodorant
Under the Arm
Each Day.**

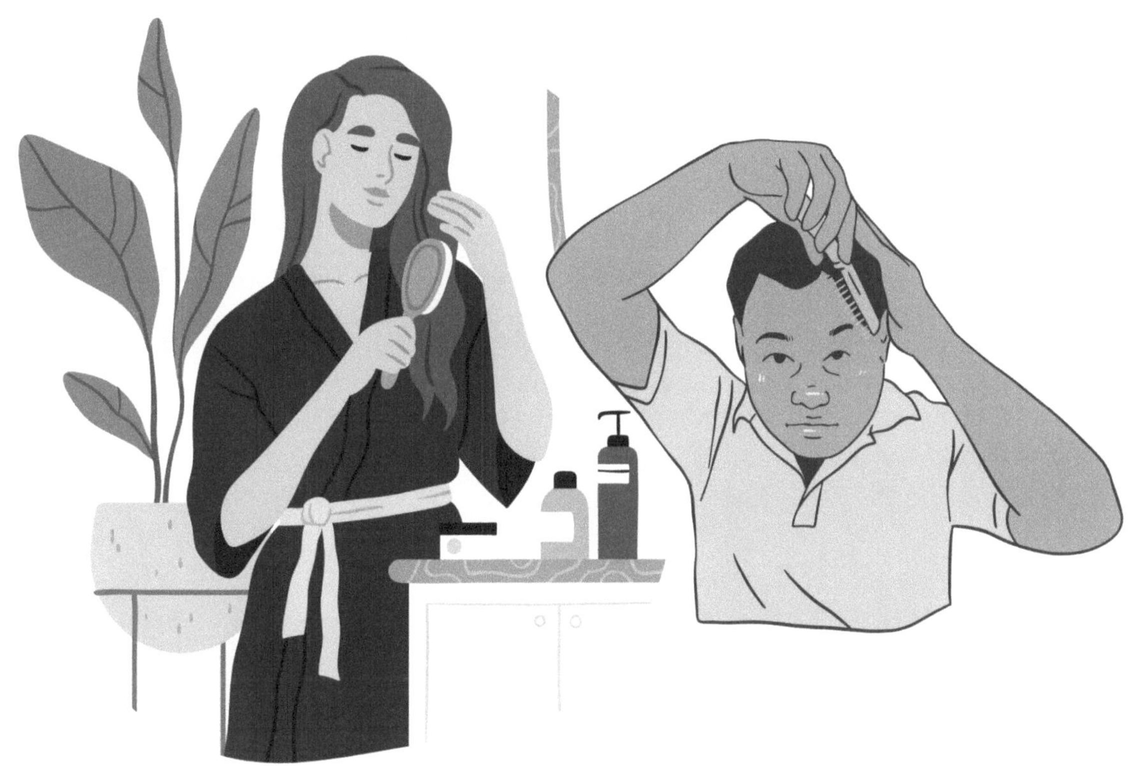

Brush or comb hair every day

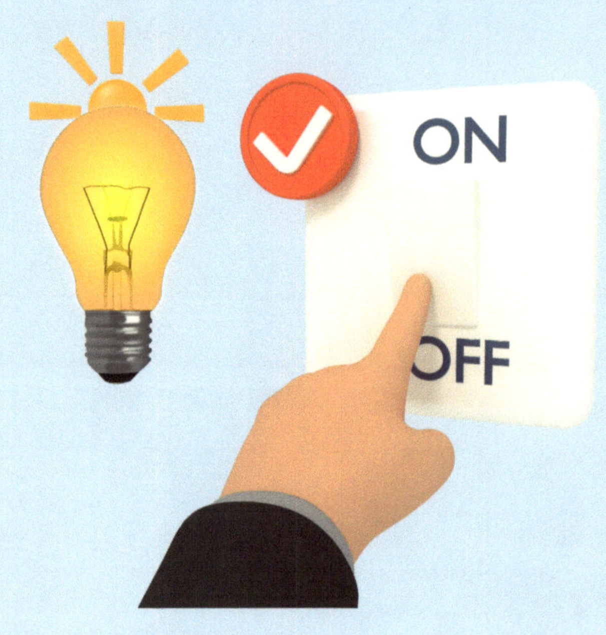

Turn lights Off when not needed

MAKE SURE YOUR HANDS ARE DRY

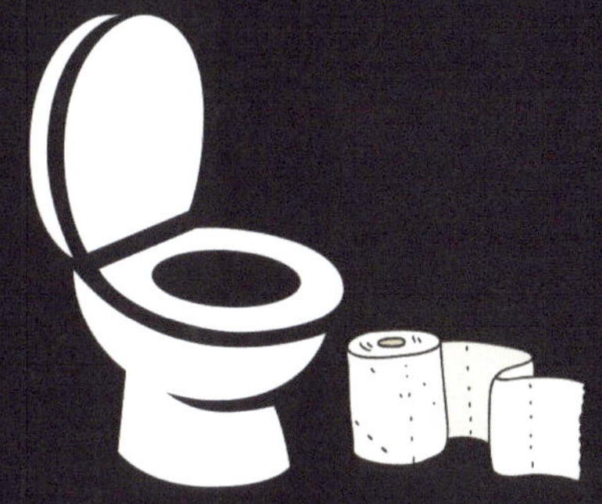
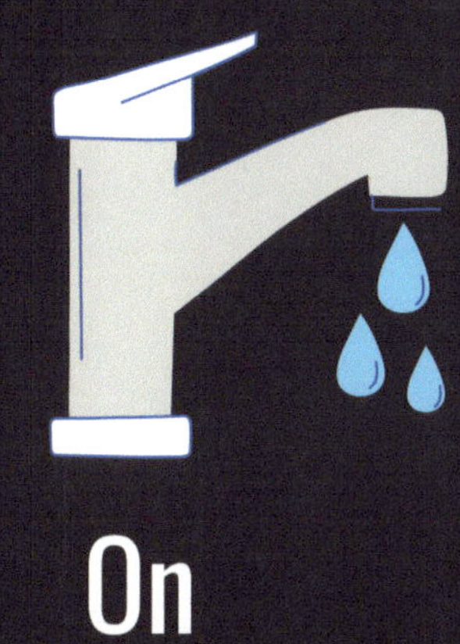

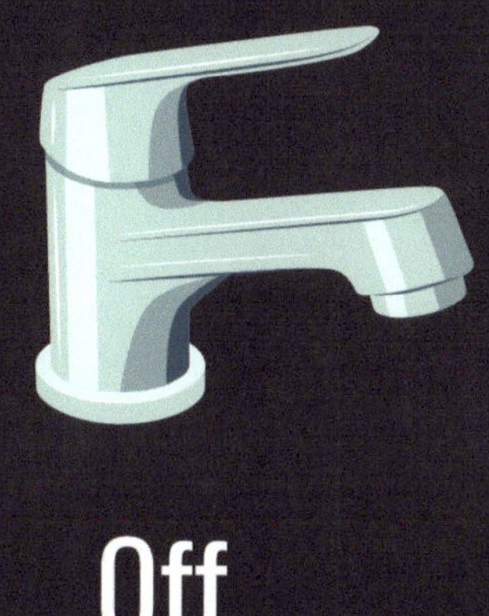

Wash hands after using toilet

Dry Hands

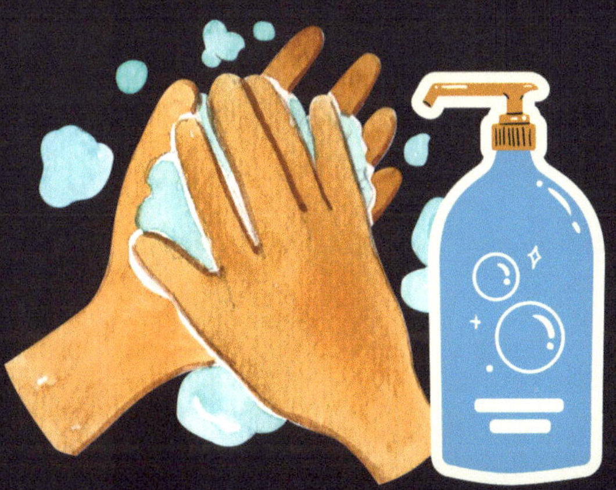
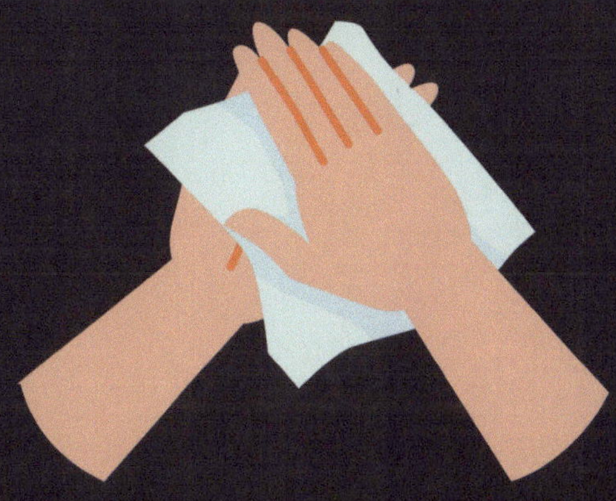

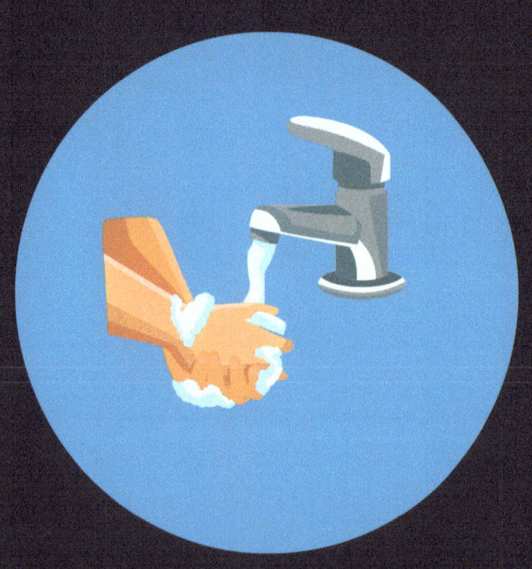

Wash hands before handling food

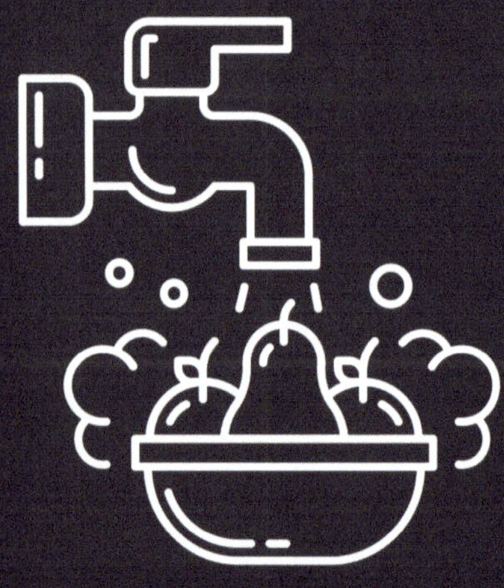

Wash fruit and vegetables

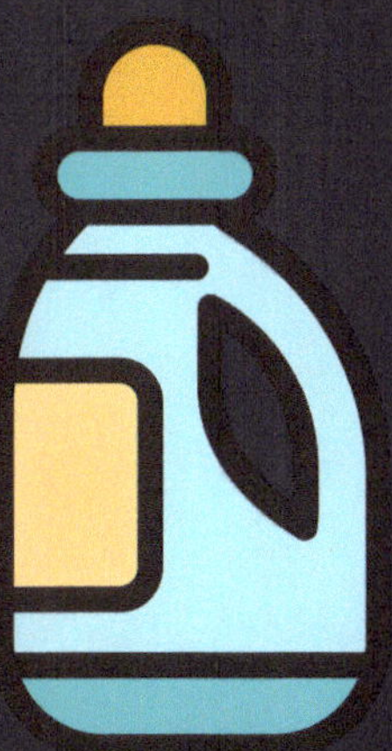

Washing Solution to remove stains Fill cap put in washing machine draw.

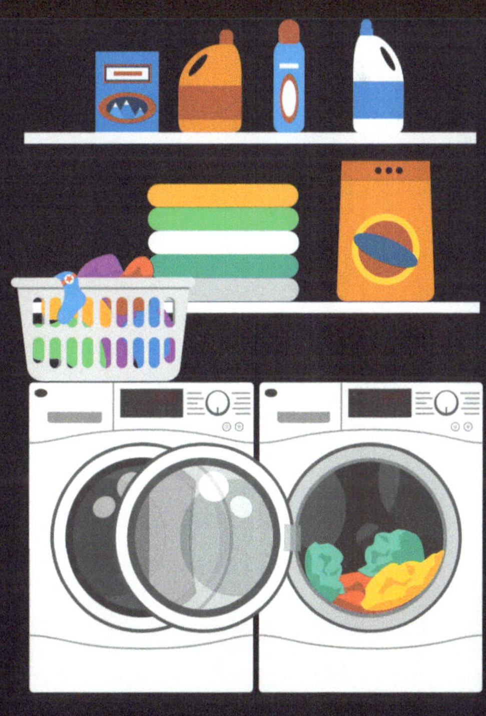

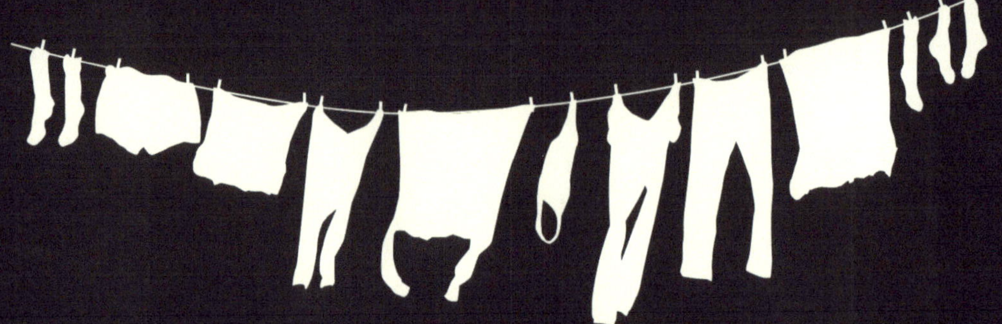
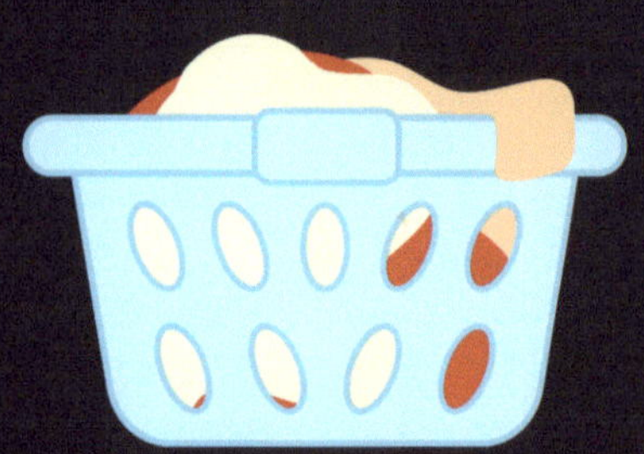

Dry Clothes

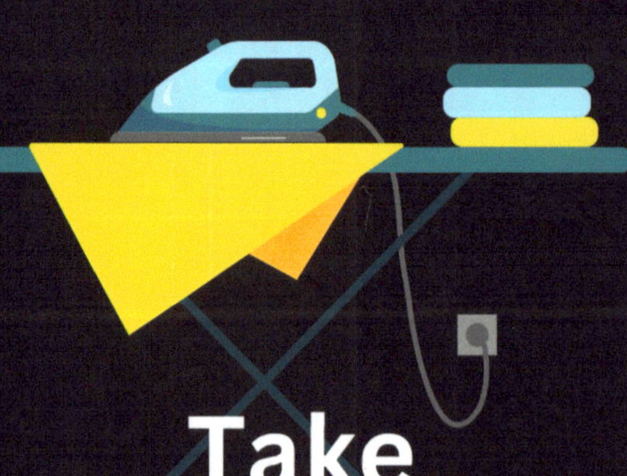

Turn iron off
after ironing
Take
plug out.

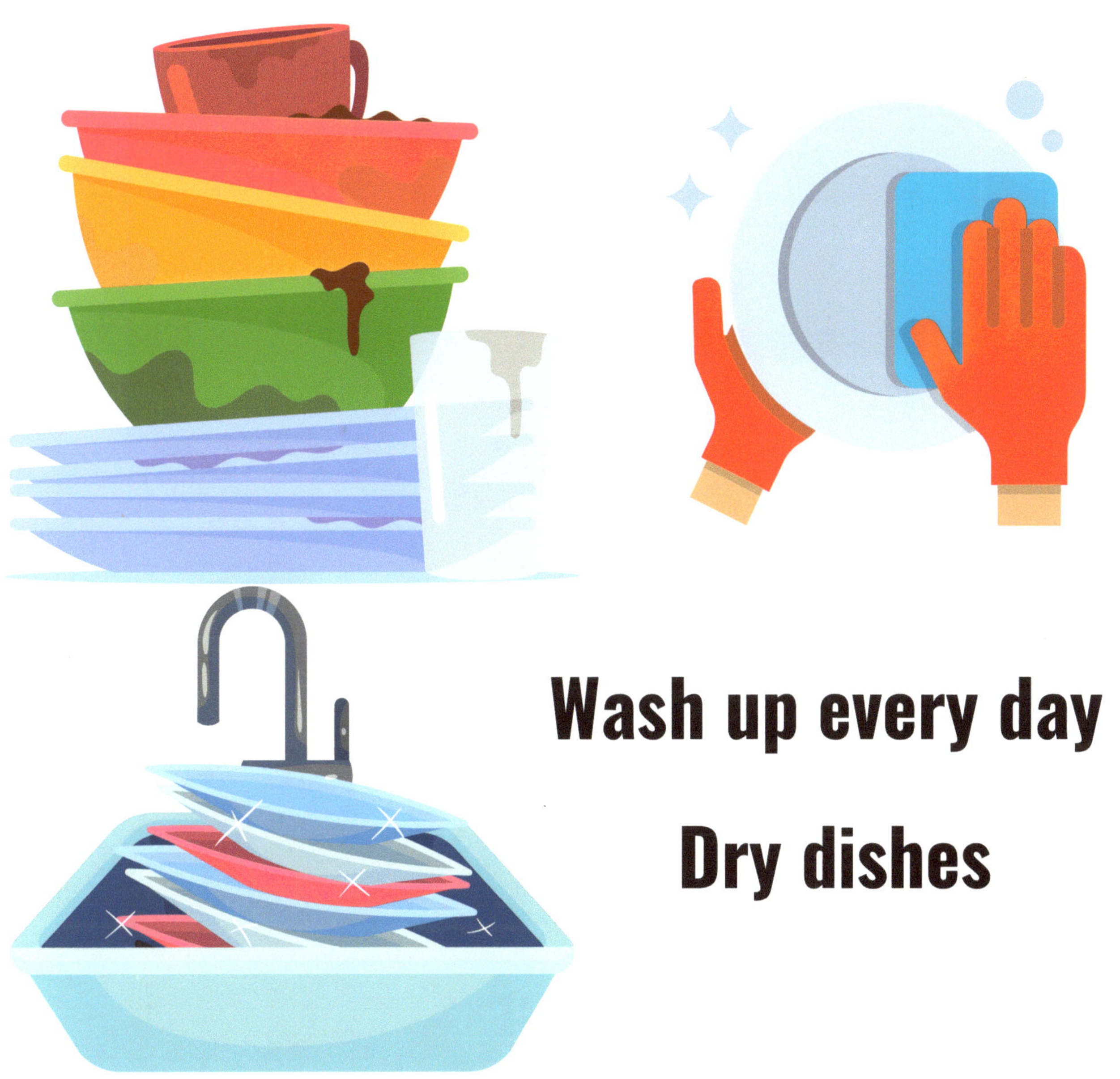

Wash up every day

Dry dishes

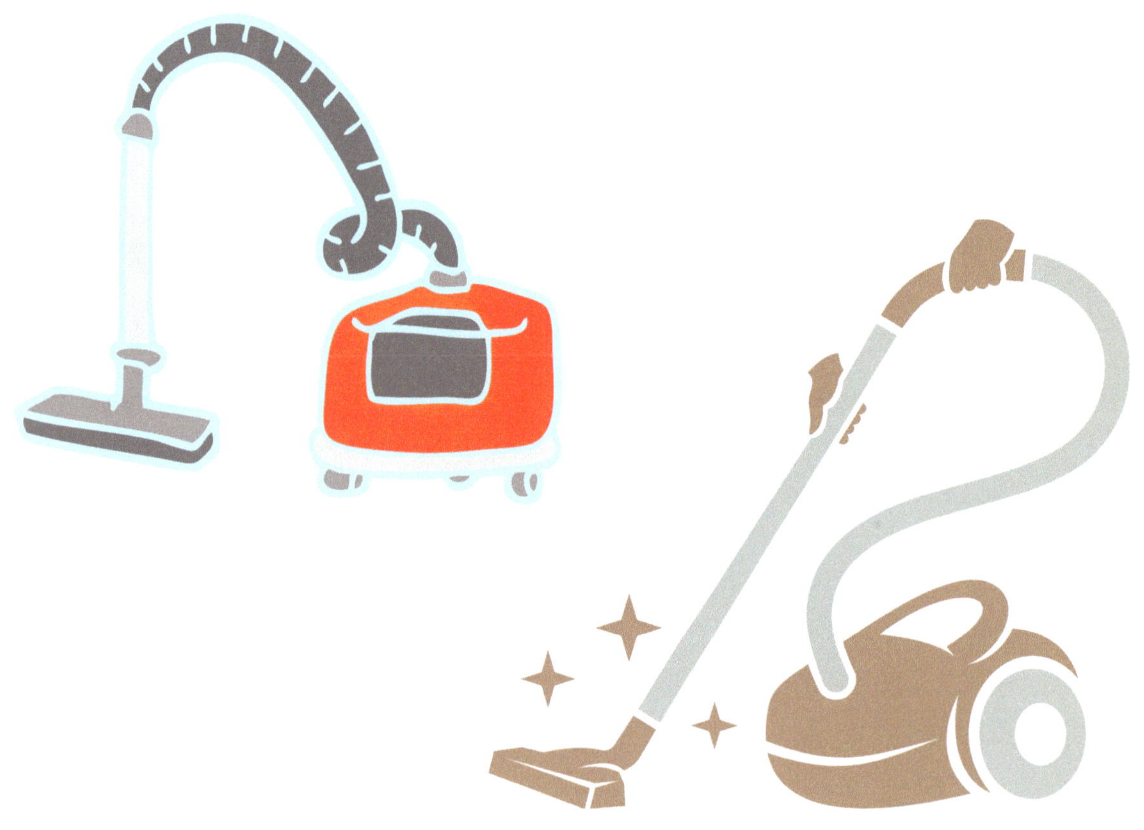

Hoover
Floor

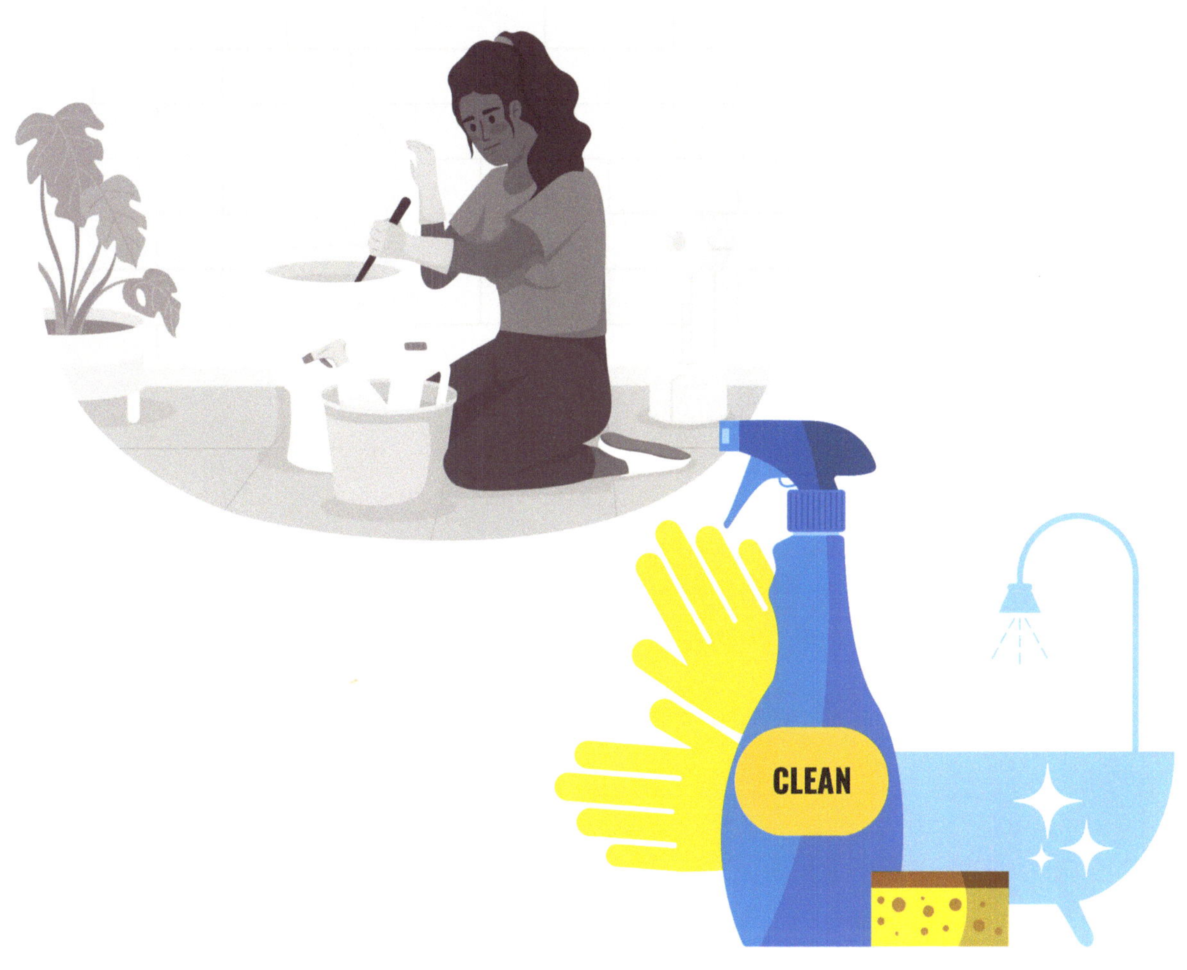

Clean Bathroom Regularly

**Lock door
Take key with you.**

Keep phone
charged

Take phone
with you.

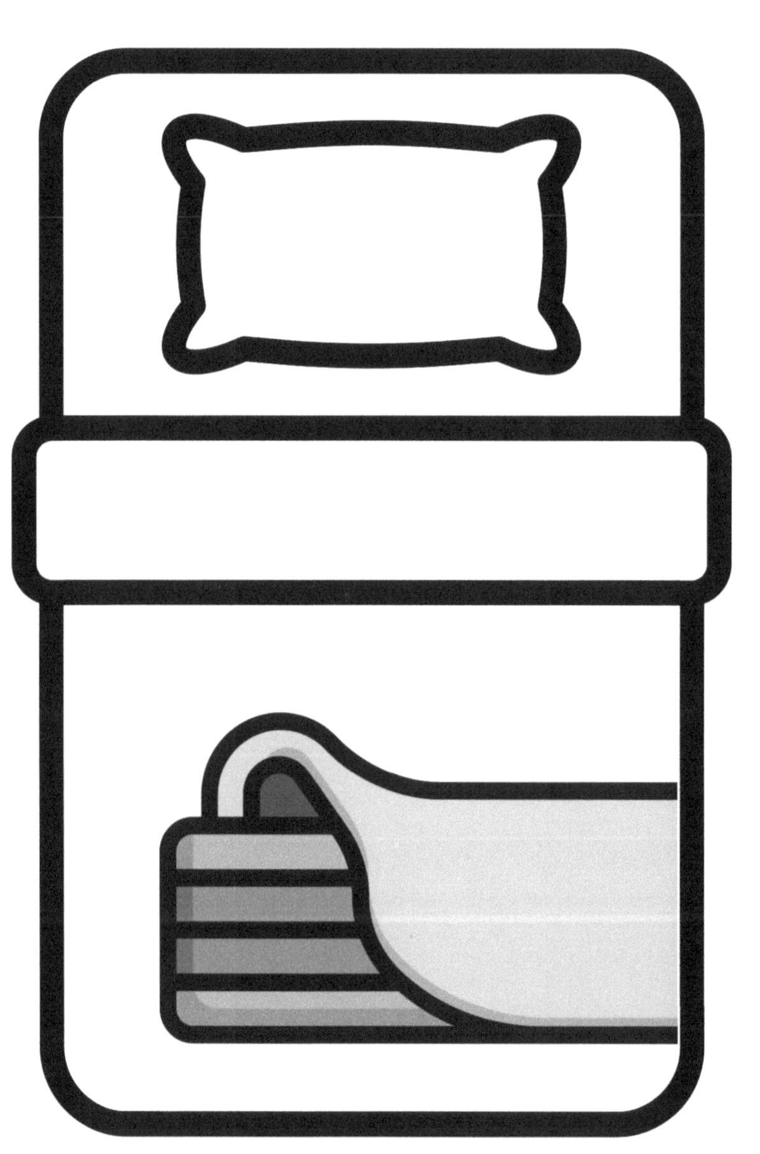

Change
bed sheets
and
Duvet Cover
Once a Week

Wash in
Washing
Machine

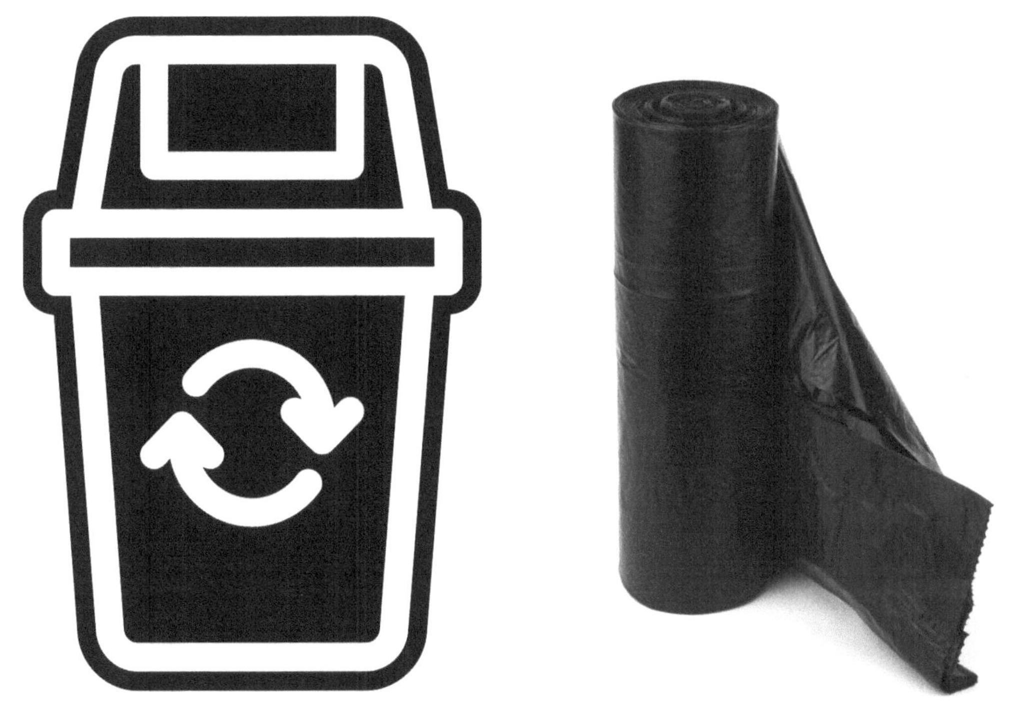

**Put black bin liner in
bin every time you empty**

Empty bin
stop flies

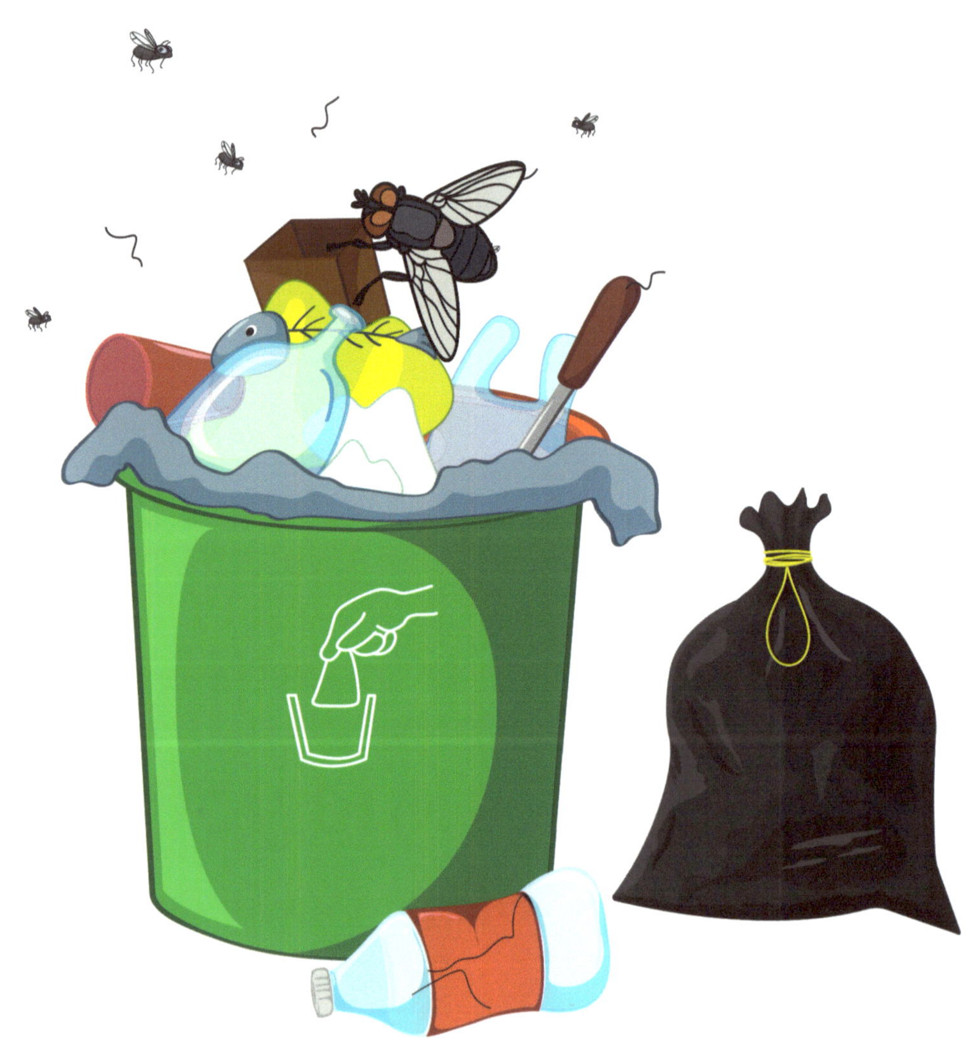

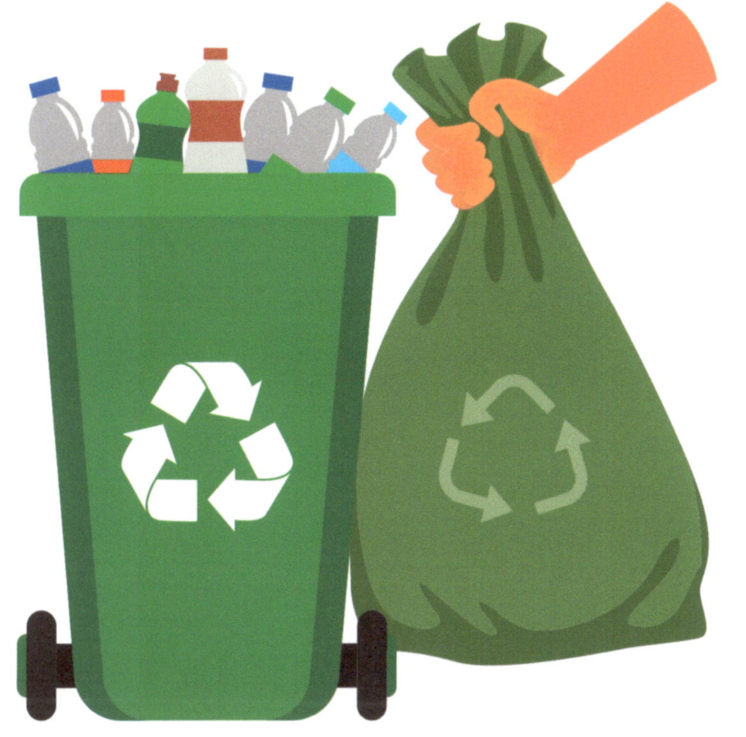

Put Plastics
and cardboard
in different
outside bin

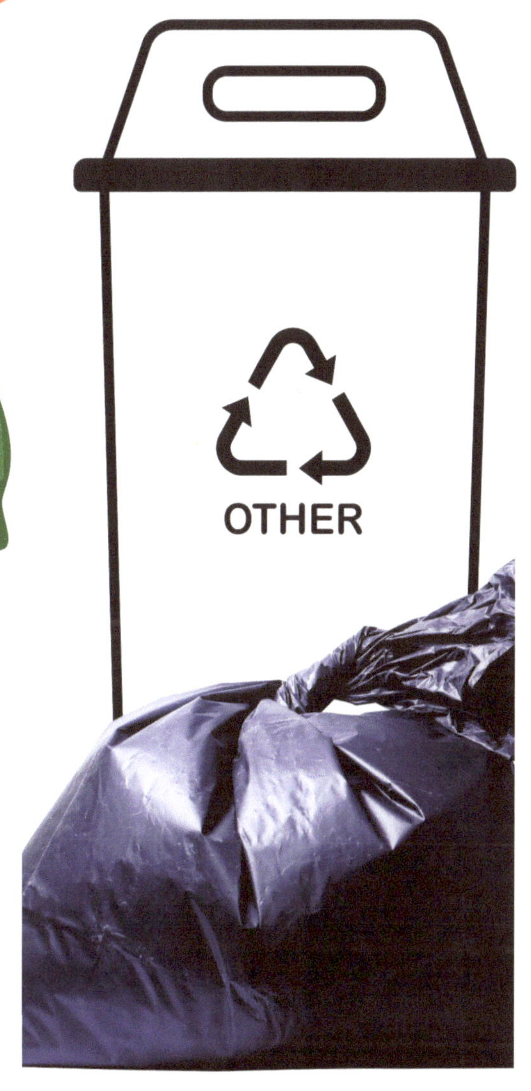

OTHER

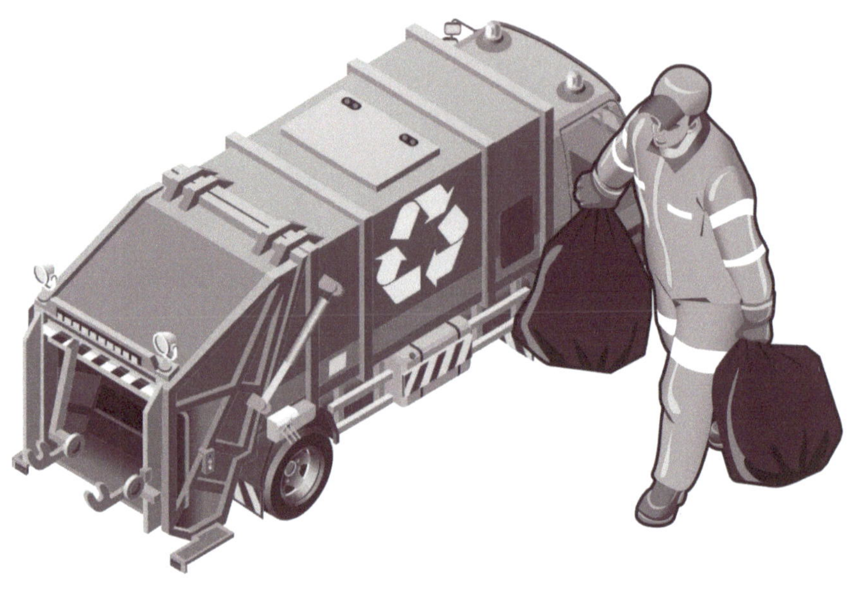

Leave bins out to be picked up.

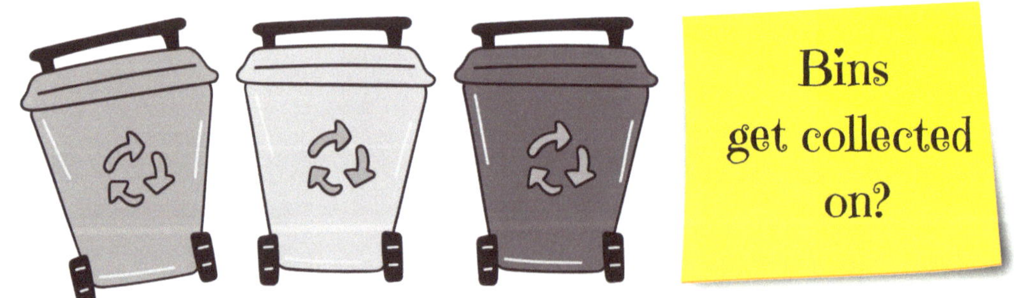

Write note of bin day

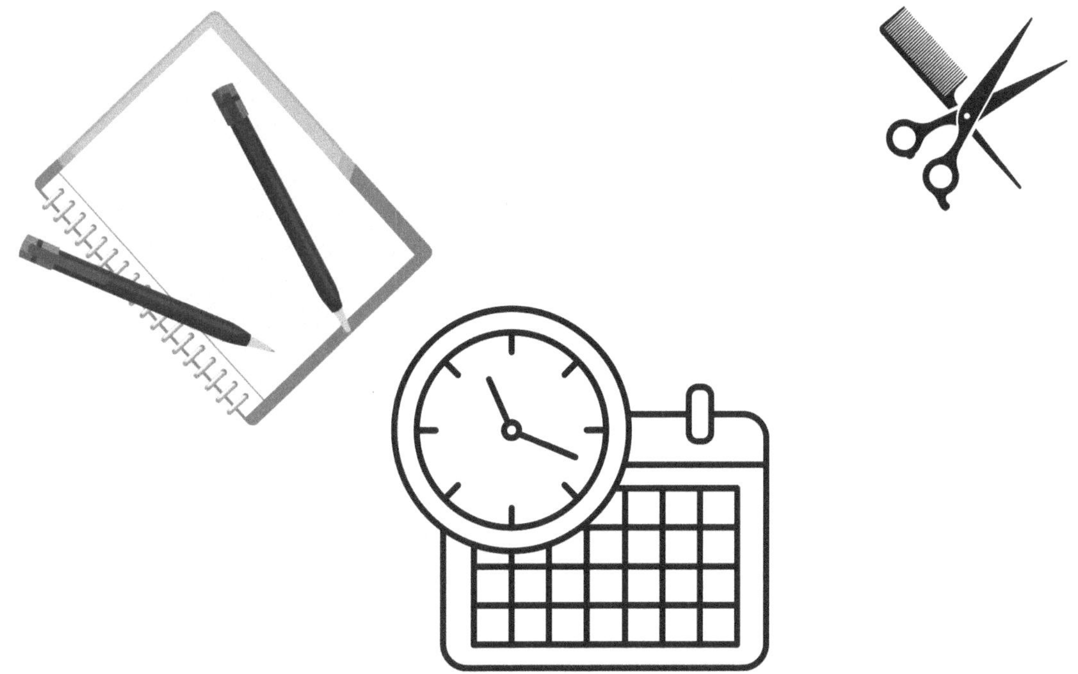

Write down Appointments

www.ingramcontent.com/pod-product-compliance
Lightning Source LLC
Chambersburg PA
CBHW040051240726
48664CB00004B/1152